PATIENT'S GUIDE TO RETINAL AND OPTIC NERVE STEM CELL SURGERY

Jeffrey N. Weiss, M.D.

Copyright (c) 2014 by Jeffrey N. Weiss, M.D.

FOR ALL OUR PATIENTS

PATIENT'S GUIDE TO RETINAL AND OPTIC NERVE STEM CELL SURGERY

WHY DID I WRITE THIS BOOK?

I am the Principal Investigator of a study performing surgery for untreatable retinal and optic nerve conditions. When performing a new surgery for an untreatable condition, it is very important for the patient to fully understand the possible benefits and the risks of the procedure.

While it may be presumptuous to say, patient's participating in such a study always have a choice. That choice is to participate or not to participate. When patients come to my office, I always conclude my explanation of the surgery with the statement, "If you have any misgivings with what I have told you, then do not undergo the procedure. I would rather we part as friends then perform a procedure when you have reservations."

Patients sometimes say to me "My doctor never heard of this work." I point to my 6 telephone lines on the telephone in my examination room and suggest they invite their doctor to call me for a personal explanation. My study is listed on the National Institute of Health (NIH) website. I am available by telephone and email for any questions.

While it is impossible for a physician to know everything, in order to hold himself out as an expert for his patients, he should have an open and inquiring mind.

I believe that it is critical for physicians and patients to approach stem cell surgery fairly and scientifically. It is vital that the required tests be performed in the postoperative period and that patients adhere to follow up requirements for progress to be made.

WHY AM I DOING STEM CELL RESEARCH?

Many physicians and scientists believe that to treat the presently "untreatable" conditions and to reverse existing damage, we must use the body's own reparative and regenerative abilities. This may potentially be provided by stem cells. I hope to help advance the development of this approach which would benefit many thousands of patients in the future.

WHO IS THIS BOOK FOR?

Typically, this book will be read by the family member or friend of a patient who is losing or has already lost their vision. The patient has been to many specialists over the years, and been told that there is nothing anyone can do, while they continue to lose their vision. So, frequently they haven't been to an eye doctor in the last year or more.

SECTION 1

WHAT ARE STEM CELLS?

A cell that can reproduce and has the potential to change or differentiate into another type of cell.

HOW MANY TYPES OF STEM CELLS ARE THERE?

There are 4 basic types:

1. Embryonic

2. Parthenogenetic

3. "Adult" stem cells

4. Induced pluripotent stem cells

    EMBRYONIC CELLS are generally taken from very early fertilized embryos. They can give rise to any type of cell, but this could be a disadvantage as well, because unrestrained, they can form tumors.

    PARTHENOGENETIC CELLS are taken from unfertilized eggs. Since the eggs are not fertilized, the stem cells they produce are genetically compatible with the woman who donated the egg.

"ADULT" STEM CELLS are found in different organs, including bone marrow, fat or adipose tissue and cord blood. The name "adult" can be confusing as they are also found in fetal tissue. It is the cell that is considered "adult" not the place where it came from. Like embryonic stem cells, adult stem cells can reproduce, but less so than embryonic, and unlike embryonic cells, adult stem cells generally form cells in their own tissue type, making the chance of tumor formation much less likely.

INDUCED PLURIPOTENT STEM CELLS are differentiated cells that can be stimulated to return to an undifferentiated state. A recent Noble Prize in Medicine was awarded to a Japanese researcher who developed the method to change a skin cell into a stem cell.

HOW LONG HAVE WE KNOWN ABOUT STEM CELLS?

Researchers have been working in this field since the 1940's and the bone marrow transplant, in use for many decades to treat leukemia, can be considered an adult stem cell transplant.

****

SECTION 2

WHAT IS RESEARCH?

Research is conducted to prove, or disapprove, a hypothesis. A procedure may be "proven" to work, but may not be commonly "accepted" by most physicians. Why?" Because the procedure may be difficult or too time consuming to perform, too expensive in terms of the drugs or equipment required, or not paid for by insurance companies. Remember, insurance companies are in business to make money. They do not pay for any procedure that they consider experimental. Their definition of "experimental" is anything outside the mainstream. So anything new and not commonly performed is not normally covered.

The insurance company may ask for articles and papers and you may appeal their decision not to reimburse, but at the end of the day, they won't pay for it. I know this to be the case, having been through this process for my patients many times. Not one appeal was successful, for at the end of multiple appeals, the insurance company simply quoted the patient's insurance policy, which stated that their contract doesn't pay for experimental procedures. The process is dressed in the guise of a fair and objective hearing, but is designed to waste your time, hoping the patient or physician will eventually give up and go away as the decision not to pay was already made prior to all the appeals.

WHO PAYS FOR "RESEARCH?"

Research is paid for by grants from the Federal Government, from pharmaceutical and device companies, from private foundations and Universities, and by patients.

The pharmaceutical industry has a research and development budget nearly double that of the National Institutes of Health. Sounds good? Not really. In 1990, they spent 8.4 billion dollars on research, and 55.2 billion dollars in 2006, but fewer successful drugs have been introduced, and 75% of them are similar to already existing drugs. Only 25% offer an improvement over existing medications.

Especially now, in this time of budgetary cutbacks, only a small minority of worthwhile research grants are ever funded by the government. When funds are so limited there is political pressure to only fund studies with a pressing social impact. It may take a researcher more than a year to write a research proposal. In fact, frequently the research proposal includes the data showing that the research has already been done! The results prove the hypothesis and further funding is needed to continue the work.

Everyone, including the government, likes to "pick a winner" and this is made possible by already performing the study you are asking for the money to perform!

WHAT IS BIAS?

Pharmaceutical companies pay physicians handsomely to participate in drug research. They may pay for each patient included in the study, offer grant money for physician "research", pay honoraria for the doctor to give lectures, and pay travel expenses. The physician himself may have been given or own stock in the company. The physician is supposed to list his "financial disclosures" when presenting a paper or giving a talk.

Listing financial support doesn't eliminate bias, it just makes everyone aware of potential bias. The pharmaceutical companies pay many physicians in this manner, much like large companies contribute to both political parties, so it is commonplace to see financial disclosures. A doctor on the "payroll" will be unlikely to say something bad about the drug or instrument, or study. Physicians are people too, and as such, have the same emotions as everyone else. There is altruism, generosity, compassion, as well as jealously, envy and stubbornness.

All research, and indeed all work, has some degree of bias. The physician earns money performing treatments, and of course he wants the treatments to be successful. That is just human nature.

WHAT IS THE ROLE OF THE FDA?

The Food and Drug Administration (FDA) mission is to regulate food, drugs and medical devices and not the practice of medicine.

Medical advances come in two basic ways:

1. Large pharmaceutical companies spend many years testing drugs, and perform large studies costing many hundreds of millions of dollars. The costs are so high that only potential blockbuster drugs are allowed to run the gauntlet of clinical trials. This accounts for the decreasing number of truly new drugs to fight or prevent diseases, i.e. antibiotics and vaccines.

2. Physicians initially produce anecdotal reports but move at a much more rapid pace and self-correct via education and peer review.

The FDA has assumed authority over all stem cell transplants, with few exemptions. This was accomplished in 2006 by changing one word. The original rule spoke to cells and tissue placed " into another human." The new rule was changed to "into a human" that now means that stem cells, even your own, are now regulated by the FDA as a drug.

The effect of this regulation has been to drive investment, companies, research and jobs out of the U.S. and to other countries with less onerous regulation.

Consequently, most of the stem cell studies now listed on the National Institutes of Health website, being performed in the U.S., involve proprietary products and are supported by companies. The exceptions are those studies using the patient's own bone-marrow or adipose derived stem cells. Since these studies use the patient's own stem cells, there is no proprietary product. They are conducted under an Institutional Review Board or IRB, which is a committee of physicians, experts and lay people that insure the ethical and safe treatment of patients, and the scientific merits and validity of the proposed study.

Physician sponsored studies tend to be more quick to respond to changes. During the last 6 months our study has, in response to published articles and our own patient observation, made changes in the stem cell separation procedure and modified our surgical procedure.

WHAT DO THE DIFFERENT PHASES OF A STUDY MEAN?

Phase 1 - A new drug or treatment is given to a small group of people, for the first time, to evaluate its safety, determine a safe dosage and monitor for side effects.

Phase 2 - The drug or treatment is given to a larger group of people to determine effectiveness and safety.

Phase 3 - The drug or treatment is given to large groups of people to determine effectiveness and safety, compare it to other commonly used treatments and collect data.

Phase 4 - These are studies performed after the drug or treatment has been marketed. They are performed to determine the effectiveness in various populations and identify side effects observed with long-term use.

WHAT IS EVIDENCE BASED MEDICINE?

Evidence-based medicine is defined as "the conscientious, explicit and judicious use of current best evidence in making decisions about the care of individual patients."

The United States Preventive Services Task Force has rated evidence concerning the effectiveness of treatment.

Level 1 - Evidence obtained from a properly designed randomized controlled trial.

Level II-1 - Evidence obtained from well-designed controlled trials without randomization.

Level II-2 - Evidence obtained from a well-designed case-control or cohort study, preferably from more than one center or research group.

Level II-3 - Evidence obtained from multiple time series with or without the intervention. Dramatic results in uncontrolled trials may be considered as this level of evidence.

Level III - Opinions or reports of respected authorities or expert committees.

HOW DOES THE EYE WORK?

RETINA

The eye is like a video camera. The cornea is the clear part of the eye, overlying the iris or colored part, which focuses light through the lens of the eye that further focuses the image onto the retina. The retina is like the film in the camera.

We can divide the retina into two parts, the macula, and the peripheral retina. The macula represents approximately 5% of the retinal area, and the peripheral retina the remaining 95%. The macula is considered the center of the retina, and is associated with central vision. It allows you see tiny detail, drive a car, recognize faces and read this book. The other 95% of the retina is the peripheral retina that gives us our side vision. It allows us to notice movement "out of the corner of our eye" and is useful when walking down a street or driving an automobile so we are aware and able to notice what is around us.

OPTIC NERVE

The light hitting the retina is processed by the retina and the electrical signals sent via the optic nerve to the brain for interpretation. Anything that affects the visual pathway can affect the vision. If we think of the eye as a video camera, the optic nerve is the electric cord that runs from the camera to the video monitor, or the brain. If the camera works, but the electric cord is cut, you don't see a picture.

In this book, we are confining ourselves to studies treating retinal and optic nerve conditions.

****

SECTION 3

CONDITIONS TREATED IN STUDIES

Age-related Macular Degeneration (AMD)

AMD is a degenerative retinal disease related to age which generally begins when patients are in their 50's or early 60's and can lead to the loss of central vision. It is the leading cause of visual loss in this age group and older. AMD is typically divided into a "wet" or neovascular type and a "dry" type of AMD. The dry type may be further subdivided into typical dry AMD that may transition into the wet type and geographic atrophy. Approximately 88% of patients have the dry type and 12% the wet type of AMD, yet the wet type accounts for approximately 90% of the overall visual loss experienced by patients.

The wet type of AMD is characterized by the growth of new blood vessels under the retina, at or near the macula. These new blood vessels can leak fluid or blood leading to the loss of central vision and scarring. Injections of medicine and/or laser treatment are used to treat this condition.

Vitamins as recommended by the Age-related Eye Disease Study (AREDS) group can slow the progression of dry to wet AMD. At the present time, there is no treatment for geographic atrophy. This type of dry AMD is characterized by retinal atrophy that may be at, or around the center of vision. Patients with this condition may experience a loss of central vision or "holes" in their vision around their central vision.

Cone dystrophy

This is an inherited or genetic condition in which the cone system is predominantly affected, although the rod system may be later affected. Most cases are of autosomal dominant inheritance. Age of onset, rate of progression and severity vary. The condition may begin in childhood, midlife, or at an older age. The progression of the loss of vision is more rapid in patients with the early onset of visual symptoms. The loss of vision may not be symmetric and is seldom much below 20/200. There is no treatment at the present time.

Cone-Rod Dystrophy

Patients with this condition generally present with a loss in central and color vision and the development of night blindness. The symptoms may start early in life or even in adulthood. This condition, also termed inverse pigmentary retinal dystrophy, may be related to retinitis pigmentosa.

Retinitis Pigmentosa (rod-cone dystrophies)

These terms refer to a large spectrum of retinal disorders of variable age of onset, progression rate, severity and mode of inheritance.

"Typical" Retinitis Pigmentosa

Patients with this condition typically experience a loss of night vision in childhood or early adulthood. There is a progressive contraction of the visual field and frequently profound loss of vision in middle or later life. Usher's Syndrome is typical retinitis pigmentosa with congenital deafness. The condition may be inherited or mutational.

There are related conditions, which may represent incomplete form of RP called atypical pigmentary retinal dystrophy's which are further subdivided into different conditions.

Stargardt's Macular Dystrophy

This is the most common juvenile retinal degenerative disease. Patients present with visual loss during childhood or early adulthood, although some experience symptoms later in life. It is inherited as an autosomal recessive trait in most patients.

Optic Nerve Conditions

Anterior Ischemic Optic Neuropathy

This condition is more prevalent in men, ages 45 - 65 years old, in patients with a history of vascular disease, i.e. hypertension, diabetes mellitus, high cholesterol. It is also has an anatomical association in which the "cup" or depression in the center of the optic nerve is small.

Optic Nerve Trauma

This condition is typically seen in patients after brain tumor surgery or after other trauma like motor vehicle accidents with head trauma.

Glaucoma

This condition causes optic nerve damage and visual loss as a result of a pressure within the eye that damages the optic nerve. Generally the eye pressure is higher than what is considered normal, but sometimes the pressure may seem normal and these cases are termed "normal tension glaucoma."

****

SECTION 4

REPLACEMENT VS. RESCUE THERAPY

The retinal and subretinal environment can influence the differentiation and functionality of transplanted cells.

Transplanted cells must integrate into the surrounding tissue for replacement therapy to succeed.

Rescue refers to the preservation and hopefully the restoration of function of tissue that was destined to die or malfunction due to an underlying disease.

Transplanted cells can secrete numerous molecules that may exert a beneficial effect on the retina/choroid even if they do not cure the underlying disease.

At the present time, we do not know whether retinal or optic nerve stem cell surgery works. That is why these studies are being performed.

HOW ARE THE STEM CELLS ADMINISTERED?

RETROBULBAR - The cells are injected behind the eye into the posterior orbit or eye socket and tissues surrounding the eye.

SUBTENON - The cells are injected under one of the layers of tissue overlying the white part, or sclera, of the eye. The injection is done from the front of the eye and the material spreads under the Tenon's tissue posteriorly, towards the back of the eye.

INTRAVITREAL - The cells are injected into the vitreous cavity of the eye. Intravitreal injections are commonly performed to treat wet age-related macular degeneration.

INTRARETINAL/SUBRETINAL/INTO THE OPTIC NERVE - Prior to injecting cells into or under the retina or into the optic nerve, a vitrectomy is performed. In this procedure, small instruments are placed into the eye and the vitreous body, (the natural gel inside the eye) is removed and replaced with a clear liquid. This surgery has been performed since the 1980's. The surgeon then has access to inject cells into or under the retina or into the optic nerve.

****

DEFINITIONS

Autologous - Derived or transferred from the same individual's body. Also known as an "autograft" or "autotransplant."

Heterologous (Xenotransplant) - Derived or transferred from another species.

Homologous - Deriving from a common primitive origin.

Allograft - Tissue taken from an individual of the same species as the recipient but with different hereditary factors.

Open-label trial - Both patients and researcher know which treatment is being administered.

Single-blind trial - The patient does not know which treatment is being administered, but the researcher does.

Double-blind trial - Neither the patient nor the researcher knows what treatment is being administered.

Non-Randomized Trial - A clinical trial in which the participants choose which group they want to be in, or they are assigned to a particular treatment group by the researchers.

Randomized Trial - The participants are assigned by chance to different groups comparing different treatments. At the time of the trial, it is unknown which treatment is best. Neither the participants nor the researcher can choose the group.

Multi-Center Trial - A trial conducted at more than one center.

****

SECTION 5

CLINICALTRIALS.GOV registered studies (NATIONAL INSTITUTES OF HEALTH (NIH) WEBSITE)

Information Current as of 1/2/14

Note: The order of the listed studies is as appears on the NIH website. A lower numbered study is not meant to imply that it is somehow better than a higher numbered study. The number in parenthesis represents the study number as shown on the website. The order is discontinuous because other non-retinal stem cell studies, as well as completed studies and studies not presently with open enrollment for patients, are also listed.

The following information is taken from the NIH website from sites identified by typing "Eye Stem Cells" in the Search box. Not all studies have supplied all the information. I have, in some cases, simplified the information they provided and in other cases corrected contradictory information and spelling mistakes. I have done my best in representing the material that was provided in the "Full Text View" section of each study.

1. (1) TITLE - Stem Cell Ophthalmology Treatment Study (SCOTS)

ClinicalTrials.gov identifier: NCT01920867

OFFICIAL TITLE - Bone Marrow Derived Stem Cell Ophthalmology Treatment Study

SPONSOR - Retina Associates of South Florida

COLLABORATOR - MD Stem Cells

CONDITIONS TREATED - Age-related Macular Degeneration (Geographic Atrophy)
- Retinal Disease (Retinitis Pigmentosa, Cone-rod dystrophy, Stargardt's Macular Dystrophy
- Optic Nerve Disease

- Glaucoma

PURPOSE OF STUDY - To determine the effectiveness of autologous (from the same patient) bone marrow derived stem cells in the treatment of various retinal and optic nerve conditions

TYPE OF STUDY - Interventional

NUMBER OF PATIENTS TO BE ENROLLED - 300

STUDY SITE - Retina Associates of South Florida, Margate, Florida

PRINCIPAL INVESTIGATOR - Jeffrey N. Weiss, MD

CONTACT - Steven Levy, MD 203-423-9494

stevenlevy@mdstemcells.com

LENGTH OF STUDY - START DATE - August 2013
- END DATE - August 2017

PROCEDURE - Arm 1 - Injection of stem cells: Retrobulbar, Subtenons, Intravenous

Arm 2 - Injection of stem cells: Intravitreal, Retrobulbar, Subtenons, Intravenous

Arm 3 - A vitrectomy is performed, and the stem cells are injected under the retina, or into the optic nerve, depending on the condition treated.

DETAILED DESCRIPTION - Eyes with loss of vision from retinal or optic nerve conditions generally considered irreversible will be treated with a combination of injections of autologous bone marrow derived stem cells isolated from the bone marrow using standard medical and surgical practices. Retinal conditions may include degenerative, ischemic or physical damage (examples may include macular degeneration, hereditary retinal dystrophies such as retinitis pigmentosa, Stargardt's Macular Dystrophy, non-perfusion retinopathies, post retinal detachments.

Optic Nerve conditions may include degenerative, ischemic or physical damage (examples may include optic nerve damage from glaucoma, compression, ischemic optic neuropathy, optic atrophy).

Injections may include retrobulbar, subtenon, intravitreal, intraretinal, subretinal and intravenous. Patients will be followed for 12 months with serial comprehensive eye examinations including relevant imaging and diagnostic ophthalmic testing.

****

2. (2) TITLE - Study the Safety and Efficacy of Bone Marrow Derived Autologous Cells for the Treatment of Optic Nerve Disease (OND)

ClinicalTrials.gov identifier: NCT01834079

OFFICIAL TITLE - Study the Safety and Efficacy of Bone Marrow Derived Autologous Cells for the Treatment of Optic Nerve Disease

SPONSOR - Chaitanya Hospital, Pune, India

CONDITION TREATED - Optic Atrophy

PURPOSE OF STUDY - To determine the safety and efficacy of bone marrow derived autologous mono nuclear cell.

TYPE OF STUDY - Interventional

NUMBER OF PATIENTS TO BE ENROLLED - 24

STUDY SITE - Chaitanya Hospital, Pune, Maharashtra, India, 4

PRINCIPAL INVESTIGATOR - Anant E. Bagul, MS

CONTACT - Sachin P. Jamadar, D Ortho
8888788880
          Smita S. Bhoyar, BAMS PGCR
9372620569

LENGTH OF STUDY - START DATE - March 2011

END DATE - April 2014

PROCEDURE - Intrathecal (injection into the spinal fluid) of autologous mononuclear cells in 3 divided doses at 7 day intervals. Follow up for 3 months or as required.

DETAILED DESCRIPTION - Conditions which produce injury or dysfunction of the second cranial or optic nerve, which is generally considered a component of the central nervous system. Damage to optic nerve fibers may occur at or near their origin in the retina, at the optic disk, or in the nerve, optic chiasm, optic tract, or lateral geniculate nuclei. Clinical manifestations may include decreased visual acuity and contrast sensitivity, impaired color vision, and an afferent pupillary defect.

****

3. (3) TITLE - Clinical Trial of Autologous Bone-marrow CD34+ Stem Cells for Retinopathy

ClinicalTrials.gov Identifier: NCT01736059

OFFICIAL TITLE - A Pilot Clinical Trial of the Feasibility and Safety of Intravitreal Autologous Adult Bone Marrow Stem Cells in Treating Eyes With Vision Loss From Retinopathy

SPONSOR - University of California, Davis

CONDITIONS TREATED - Dry Age-related Macular Degeneration
Diabetic Retinopathy
Retinal Vein Occlusion
Retinitis Pigmentosa

PURPOSE OF STUDY - To determine the safety and feasibility of injecting stem cells from the bone marrow into the eye as treatment for patients who are irreversibly blind from various retinal conditions.

TYPE OF STUDY - Pilot study - Phase 1

NUMBER OF PATIENTS TO BE ENROLLED - 15

STUDY SITE - University of California, Davis

PRINCIPAL INVESTIGATOR - Susanna S. Park, MD, PhD

CONTACT - Susanna S. Park, MD PhD 916-734-6074
Marisa Salvador 916-734-6302

LENGTH OF STUDY - START DATE - July 2012
END DATE - December 2013 (Still listed as recruiting patients as of January 2014.)

PROCEDURE - Patients will undergo vitrectomy surgery with the injection of the study cells beneath the retina in the most affected eye.

DETAILED DESCRIPTION - In this pilot clinical trial, eyes with irreversible vision loss from retinal degenerative conditions (macular degeneration or retinitis pigmentosa) or retinal vascular disease (diabetic retinopathy or retinal vein occlusion) will be treated with intravitreal injection of autologous CD34+ stem cells isolated from bone marrow aspirate under Good Manufacturing Practice conditions. This study will determine whether there are any major safety and feasibility concerns using this therapy. Patients will be followed for 6 months after treatment by serial comprehensive eye examination supplemented with various retinal imaging and diagnostic tests.

****

4. (15) TITLE - Study of Human Central Nervous System Stem Cells (HuCNS-SC) in Age-related Macular Degeneration (AMD)

ClinicalTrials.gov identifier: NCT01632527

OFFICIAL TITLE - Phase 1/2 Study of the Safety and Preliminary Efficacy of Human Central Nervous System Stem Cells (HuCNS-SC) Subretinal Transplantation in Subjects With Geographic Atrophy of Age-Related Macular Degeneration

SPONSOR - StemCells, Inc.

STUDY DIRECTOR - Stephen Huhn, MD
StemCells, Inc.

CONTACT - Jocelyn Rojas, RN 510-456-4136
jocelyn.rojas@stemcellsinc.com

CONDITION TREATED - Dry Age-Related Macular Degeneration (Geographic Atrophy)

PURPOSE OF STUDY - To determine the safety and preliminary efficacy of the Company's proprietary product, purified human neural stem cells (HuCNS-SC).

TYPE OF STUDY - Open label, dose-escalation study, phase 1/2

NUMBER OF PATIENTS TO BE ENROLLED - 16

STUDY SITES - Byers Eye Institute, Stanford Hospital and Clinics, Palo Alto, California
Principal Investigator, Theodore Leng, MD
Contact - Lorella Cavael
650-498-4486
lcabael@stanford.edu
Ted Leng, MD
650-498-4486

New York Eye and Ear Infirmary, New York, New York
Principal Investigator,

Richard Rosen, MD
Contact - Katy Tai, CCRC
212-979-4251
ktai@nyeee.edu

Retina Foundation of the Southwest, Dallas, Texas
Principal Investigator, David Birch, Phd
Contact - Kirsten Locke, RN
214-363-3911 ext 114
kglocke@retinafoundation.org

LENGTH OF STUDY - START DATE - June 2012
                             END DATE - June 2014

PROCEDURE - Patients will undergo vitrectomy surgery with the injection of the study cells beneath the retina in the most affected eye. Immunosuppressive agents are orally administered for 3 months after surgery.

DETAILED DESCRIPTION - The study is an open-label dose-escalation investigation of the safety and preliminary efficacy of unilateral subretinal transplantation of HuCNS-SC cells in subjects with Geographic Atrophy secondary to Age-Related Macular Degeneration. There are 2 cohorts receiving a different amount of cells. Immunosuppressive agents will be orally administered for 3 months after surgery. Evaluations will be performed at pre-determined intervals over a one-year period with follow-up over an additional four years.

****

5. (17) TITLE - Safety and Tolerability of Sub-retinal Transplantation of Human Embryonic Stem Cell Derived Retinal Pigmented Epithelial (hESC-RPE) Cells in Patients with Stargardt's Macular Dystrophy (SMD)

ClinicalTrials.gov identifier: NCT01345006

OFFICIAL TITLE - A Phase 1/2 Open-Label, Multi-Center, Prospective Study to Determine the Safety and Tolerability of Sub-retinal Transplantation of Human Embryonic Stem Cell Derived Retinal Pigmented Epithelial (hESC-RPE) Cells in Patients with Stargardt's Macular Dystrophy (SMD)

SPONSOR - Advanced Cell Technology

CONDITION TREATED - Stargardt's Macular Dystrophy (SMD)

PURPOSE OF STUDY - To determine the safety and tolerability of the Company's proprietary product, human embryonic derived retinal pigment epithelial cells. To evaluate potential efficacy endpoints to be used in future studies of cellular therapy.

TYPE OF STUDY - Interventional study, Phase 1/2

NUMBER OF PATIENTS TO BE ENROLLED - 16

STUDY SITES - NHS Lothian Princess Alexandra Eye Pavilion Edinburgh, United Kingdom
Principal Investigator Baljean Dhillon, BMed Sci, BM, BS, FRCS
Contact - Margareet MacDonald 0131 536 3340
margaret.macdonald@luht.scot.nhs.uk

Moorfields Eye Hospital (SMD) London, England
Principal Investigator, James Bainbridge, MA, MB, BChir, Phd, FRCOphth
Contact - Heather Kneale 44(0) 207 608 4023
mol.therapy@ucl.ac.uk

LENGTH OF STUDY - START DATE - November 2011
END DATE - April 2014

PROCEDURE - Patients will undergo vitrectomy surgery with the injection of the study cells beneath the retina in the most affected eye.

DETAILED DESCRIPTION - This study is a Phase 1/2, open-label, non randomized, sequential, multi-center clinical trial. There are 5 cohorts of patients. The day of cell implantation is Day 0, and patients will remain in the study until the last visit at 12 months.

****

6. (19) TITLE - Study to Assess the Safety and Effects of Cells Injected Intravitreal in Dry Macular Degeneration

ClinicalTrials.gov identifier: NCT02024269

OFFICIAL TITLE - An Open-label, Non-Randomized, Multi-Center Study to Assess the Safety and Effects of Autologous Adipose-Derived Stromal Cells Injected Intravitreal in Dry Macular Degeneration

SPONSOR - Bioheart, Inc.

CONDITION TREATED - Dry Macular Degeneration

PURPOSE OF STUDY - To determine the efficacy of adipose derived stem cells in the treatment of dry macular degeneration

TYPE OF STUDY - Interventional study

NUMBER OF PATIENTS TO BE ENROLLED - 100

STUDY SITE - Hollywood Eye Institute, Cooper City, Florida

CONTACT - Kristin Comella 954-835-1500
kcomella@bioheartinc.com

LENGTH OF STUDY - START DATE - December 2013

END DATE - June 2016

PROCEDURE - Patients will undergo liposuction and the adipose tissue is processed to isolate the stem cells. The stem cells will then be injected intravitreal into the eye.

DETAILED DESCRIPTION - Not Supplied

****

7. (26) TITLE - Safety and Tolerability of Sub-retinal Transplantation of hESC Derived RPE (MA09-hRPE) Cells in Patients with Advanced Dry Age-Related Macular Degeneration (Dry AMD)

ClinicalTrials.gov identifier: NCT01344993

OFFICIAL TITLE - A Phase 1/2, Open-Label, Multi-Center, Prospective Study to Determine the Safety and Tolerability of Sub-retinal Transplantation of Human Embryonic Stem Cell Derived Retinal Pigmented Epithelial (MA09-hRPE) Cells in Patients with Advanced Dry AMD.

SPONSOR - Advanced Cell Technology

CONDITIONS TREATED - Age-related Macular Degeneration (AMD)

PURPOSE OF STUDY - To determine the safety and preliminary efficacy of the Company's proprietary product, human embryonic derived retinal pigment epithelial cells

TYPE OF STUDY - Open label, dose-escalation study, Phase 1/2

NUMBER OF PATIENTS TO BE ENROLLED - 16

STUDY SITES - Jules Stein Eye Institute, Los Angeles, California
Principal Investigator - Steven Schwartz, MD
Contact - Logan Hitchcock 310-825-3046

Bascom-Palmer Eye Institute, Miami, Florida
Principal Investigator - Philip Rosenfeld, MD, PhD
Contact - Cristy M Lage-Rodriguez, MS, CCRC 305-326-6117 CLage@med.miami.edu

Massachusetts Eye and Ear Infirmary, Boston, Massachusetts
Principal Investigator, Dean Elliot, MD
Jacqueline Sullivan 617-573-3920
jacqueline_sullivan@meei.harvard.edu

Wills Eye Institute, Philadelphia, Pennsylvania
Principal Investigator, Carl Regillo, MD
Contact - Shellie Markun
research@midatlanticretina.com

LENGTH OF STUDY - START DATE - April 2011
                            END DATE   - July 2014

PROCEDURE - Patients will undergo vitrectomy surgery with the injection of the study cells beneath the retina in the most affected eye.

DETAILED DESCRIPTION - This study is a Phase 1/2, open-label, non randomized, sequential, multi-center clinical trial. There are 5 cohorts of patients. The day of cell implantation is Day 0, and patients will remain in the study until the last visit at 12 months.

....

8. (27) TITLE - Safety and Tolerability of Sub-retinal Transplantation of Human Embryonic Stem Cell Derived Retinal Pigmented Epithelial (hESC-RPE) Cells in Patients with Stargardt's Macular Dystrophy (SMD)

ClinicalTrials.gov identifier: NCT01345006

OFFICIAL TITLE - A Phase 1/2 Open-Label, Multi-Center, Prospective Study to Determine the Safety and Tolerability of Sub-retinal Transplantation of Human Embryonic Stem Cell Derived Retinal Pigmented Epithelial (hESC-RPE) Cells in Patients with Stargardt's Macular Dystrophy (SMD)

SPONSOR - Advanced Cell Technology

CONDITION TREATED - Stargardt's Macular Dystrophy (SMD)

PURPOSE OF STUDY - To determine the safety and tolerability of the Company's proprietary product, human embryonic derived retinal pigment epithelial cells. To evaluate potential efficacy endpoints to be used in future studies of cellular therapy.

TYPE OF STUDY - Interventional study, Phase 1/2

NUMBER OF PATIENTS TO BE ENROLLED - 16

STUDY SITES - Jules Stein Eye Institute, Los Angeles, California
Principal Investigator - Steven Schwartz, MD
Contact - Logan Hitchcock 310-825-3046

Bascom-Palmer Eye Institute Miami, Florida
Principal Investigator, Philip Rosenfeld, MD, PhD
Contact - Alexis Morante, MS 305-482-5186
AMorante@med.miami.edu
Wills Eye Institute, Philadelphia, Pennsylvania
Principle Investigator, Carl Regillo, MD

Contact - Shellie Markun
research@midatlanticretina.com

LENGTH OF STUDY - START DATE - April 2011
END DATE - January 2014

PROCEDURE - Patients will undergo vitrectomy surgery with the injection of the study cells beneath the retina in the most affected eye.

DETAILED DESCRIPTION - This study is a Phase 1/2, open-label, non randomized, sequential, multi-center clinical trial. There are 5 cohorts of patients. The day of cell implantation is Day 0, and patients will remain in the study until the last visit at 12 months.

....

9. (29) TITLE - Autologous Bone Marrow-Derived Stem Cells Transplantation for Retinitis Pigmentosa (RETICELL)

ClinicalTrials.gov identifier: NCT01560715

OFFICIAL TITLE - Phase 2 Study of Autologous Bone Marrow-Derived Stem Cells Transplantation For Retinitis Pigmentosa

SPONSOR - University of Sao Paulo, Brazil

CONDITION TREATED - Retinitis Pigmentosa

PURPOSE OF STUDY - To evaluate the short-term safety and efficacy of a single intravitreal injection of autologous bone marrow stem cell in patients with retinitis pigmentosa

TYPE OF STUDY - Interventional - Phase 2

NUMBER OF PATIENTS TO BE ENROLLED - 50

STUDY SITE - University of Sao Paulo, Brazil

PRINCIPAL INVESTIGATOR - Rubens C Siqueira, MD, PhD

CONTACT - Rubens C Siqueira, MD, PhD
55(17)32140896

LENGTH OF STUDY - START DATE - June 2011
                  END DATE   - June 2013
(Still listed as recruiting patients as of January 2014.)

PROCEDURE - Patients will undergo one intravitreal injection of autologous bone marrow derived stem cells.

DETAILED DESCRIPTION - One intravitreal injection of a 0.1 ml cell suspension of bone marrow mononuclear stem cells under topical anesthesia.

****

10. (34) TITLE - Effect of Intravitreal Bone Marrow Stem Cells on Ischemic Retinopathy (RetinaCell)

ClinicalTrials.gov identifier: NCT01518842

OFFICIAL TITLE - Effect of Intravitreal Bone Marrow Stem Cells on Ischemic Retinopathy

SPONSOR - University of Sao Paulo, Brazil

CONDITION TREATED - Retinitis Pigmentosa

PURPOSE OF STUDY - This study aims to evaluate the behavior of the intravitreal use of bone marrow derived stem cells in patients with ischemic retinopathy.

TYPE OF STUDY - Interventional - Phase 1/2

NUMBER OF PATIENTS TO BE ENROLLED - 30

STUDY SITE - University of Sao Paulo, Brazil

PRINCIPAL INVESTIGATOR - Rubens C Siqueira, MD, PhD

CONTACT - Rubens C Siqueira, MD, PhD
55(17)32140896

LENGTH OF STUDY - START DATE - September 2011
END DATE - September 2012 (Still listed as recruiting patients as of January 2014.)

PROCEDURE - Patients will undergo one intravitreal injection of autologous bone marrow derived stem cells.

DETAILED DESCRIPTION - One intravitreal injection of a 0.1 ml cell suspension of bone marrow mononuclear stem cells under topical anesthesia.

....

11. (41) TITLE - Cell Collection to Study Retinal Diseases

ClinicalTrials.gov identifier: NCT01432847

OFFICIAL TITLE - Generation of Induced Pluripotent Stem (iPS) Cell Lines From Somatic Cells of Participants With Retinal Disease and From Somatic Cells of Matched Controls

SPONSOR - National Eye Institute

CONDITIONS STUDIED - Best Vitelliform Dystrophy (Best disease), Late-Onset Retinal Degeneration (L-ORD), and Age-Related Macular Degeneration (AMD)

PURPOSE OF STUDY - To collect hair, skin, and blood samples to study three eye disease that effect the retina: Best disease, L-ORD, and AMD.

TYPE OF STUDY - Observational

NUMBER OF PATIENTS TO BE ENROLLED - 350

STUDY SITE - National Institutes of Health Clinical Center, 9000 Rockville Pike, Bethesda, Maryland

PRINCIPAL INVESTIGATOR - Brian P Brooks, MD National Eye Institute

CONTACT - Allison T Bamji, RN   301-451-3437
bamjia@nei.nih.gov
　　　　　　　Brian P Brooks, MD   301-496-3577
brooksb@nei.nih.gov

LENGTH OF STUDY - START DATE - August 2011

END DATE - No end date listed. Still listed as recruiting patients as of January 2014.

PROCEDURE - Patients will be screened with a medical and eye disease history and undergo an eye examination. Study participants will provide a hair sample, a blood sample, and a skin biopsy. The hair will be collected from the back of the head, and the skin will be collected from the inside of the upper arm.

DETAILED DESCRIPTION - See Above. One visit to the National Eye Institute is required.

****

12. (66) TITLE - Feasibility and Safety of Adult Human Bone Marrow-derived Mesenchymal Stem Cells by Intravitreal Injection in Patients with Retinitis Pigmentosa

ClinicalTrials.gov identifier: NCT01531348

OFFICIAL TITLE - Feasibility and Safety of Adult Human Bone Marrow-Derived Mesenchymal Stem

Cells by Intravitreal Injection in Patients with Retinitis Pigmentosa

SPONSOR - Mahidol University, Ministry of Health, Thailand

CONDITIONS STUDIED - Retinitis Pigmentosa

PURPOSE OF STUDY - To determine the feasibility and safety of adult human bone marrow-derived mesenchymal stem cells by intravitreal injection in patients with retinitis pigmentosa.

TYPE OF STUDY - Observational, phase 1

NUMBER OF PATIENTS TO BE ENROLLED - 10, BY INVITATION ONLY

STUDY SITE - Siriraj Hospital Mahidol University, Bangkoknoi, Bangkok, Thailand

PRINCIPAL INVESTIGATOR - La-ongsri Atchaneeyasakul, MD Siriraj Hospital, Mahidol University

CONTACT - Not Listed

LENGTH OF STUDY - START DATE - February 2012
                  END DATE   - March 2014

PROCEDURE - An intravitreal injection of bone marrow-derived mesenchymal stem cell will be performed.

DETAILED DESCRIPTION - See Above.

****

13. (82) TITLE - Safety Study of Use of Autologous Bone Marrow Derived Stem Cell in Treatment of Age Related Macular Degeneration

ClinicalTrials.gov identifier: NCT02016508

OFFICIAL TITLE - Intravitreal Injection of Human Bone Marrow Derived Mesenchymal Stem Cell in Patients With Dry Age-related Macular Degeneration (AMD)

SPONSOR - Al-Azhar University, Nasr City, Egypt
CONDITIONS STUDIED - Dry Age-related Macular Degeneration

PURPOSE OF STUDY - To determine the feasibility and safety of adult human bone marrow-derived mesenchymal stem cells by intravitreal injection in patients with retinitis pigmentosa.

TYPE OF STUDY - Interventional

NUMBER OF PATIENTS TO BE ENROLLED - 1 (1 is listed on the website)

STUDY SITE - Al-Azhar University Medical School (Benin-Cairo) Ophthalmology Department, Cairo, Nasr City, Egypt

PRINCIPAL INVESTIGATOR - Abdelhakim Mohamed Safwat, MD

CONTACT - Abdelhakim Mohamed Safwat, MD
+201005151919
abdelhakimsafwat@gmail.com

LENGTH OF STUDY - START DATE - March 2013
END DATE - June 2015

PROCEDURE - An intravitreal injection of autologous bone marrow-derived stem cells will be performed.

DETAILED DESCRIPTION - See Above.

****

14. (88) TITLE - A Phase 1/2a, Open-Label, Single-Center, Prospective Study to Determine the Safety and Tolerability of Sub-retinal Transplantation of Human Embryonic Stem Cell Derived Retinal Pigmented Epithelial (MA09-hRPE) Cells in Patients With Advanced Dry Age-related Macular Degeneration (AMD)

ClinicalTrials.gov identifier: NCT01674829

OFFICIAL TITLE - A Phase 1/2a, Open-Label, Single-Center, Prospective Study to Determine the Safety and Tolerability of Sub-retinal Transplantation of Human Embryonic Stem Cell Derived Retinal Pigmented Epithelial (MA09-hRPE) Cells in Patients With Advanced Dry Age-related Macular Degeneration (AMD)

SPONSOR - CHA Bio & Diostech

CONDITIONS STUDIED - Advanced Dry Age-related Macular Degeneration

PURPOSE OF STUDY - To evaluate the safety and tolerability of MA09-hRPE cellular therapy in patients with advanced dry AMD. To evaluate the safety of the surgical procedures when used to implant MA09-hRPE cells. To assess the number of hRPE cells to be transplanted in future studies. To evaluate on an exploratory basis potential efficacy endpoints to be used in future studies of MA09-hRPE cellular therapy.

TYPE OF STUDY - Interventional, phase 1/2a

NUMBER OF PATIENTS TO BE ENROLLED - 12

STUDY SITE - CHA Bundang Medical Center, Seongnam-si, Gyeonggi-do, Republic of Korea

PRINCIPAL INVESTIGATOR - Wonkyung Song, MD, PhD CHA Bundang Medical Center

CONTACT - Wonkyung Song, MD, PhD 82-31-780-5479

LENGTH OF STUDY - START DATE - September 2012
END DATE - April 2016

PROCEDURE - Not Provided

DETAILED DESCRIPTION - 4 groups with escalating doses of stem cells. Further details not provided.

****

15. (90) TITLE - Safety and Tolerability of MA09-hRPE Cells in Patients With Stargardt's Macular Dystrophy (SMD)

ClinicalTrials.gov identifier: NCT01625559

OFFICIAL TITLE - A Phase 1, Open-Label, Prospective Study to Determine the Safety and Tolerability of Sub-retinal Transplantation of Human Embryonic Stem Cell Derived Retinal Pigmented Epithelial (MA09-hRPE) Cells in Patients With Stargardt's Macular Dystrophy (SMD)

SPONSOR - CHA Bio & Diostech

CONDITIONS STUDIED - Stargardt's Macular Dystrophy (SMD)

PURPOSE OF STUDY - To evaluate the safety and tolerability of MA09-hRPE cellular therapy in patients with SMD. To evaluate the safety of the surgical procedures when used to implant MA09-hRPE cells. To assess the number of hRPE cells to be transplanted in future studies. To optimize the dose of cells to be used in future studies of MA09-hRPE cellular therapy.

TYPE OF STUDY - Interventional, phase 1

NUMBER OF PATIENTS TO BE ENROLLED - 3

STUDY SITE - CHA Bundang Medical Center, Seongnam-si, Gyeonggi-do, Republic of Korea

PRINCIPAL INVESTIGATOR - Wonkyung Song, MD, PhD CHA Bundang Medical Center

CONTACT - Wonkyung Song, MD, PhD 82-31-780-5479

LENGTH OF STUDY - START DATE - September 2012
- END DATE - October 2014

PROCEDURE - Not Provided

DETAILED DESCRIPTION - Further details not provided.

****
****

www.ingramcontent.com/pod-product-compliance
Lightning Source LLC
Chambersburg PA
CBHW040919180526
45159CB00002BA/530